Lean Waist Warrior

Meal Plan

With Shopping list

By

R.S Jacobs

www.leanwaistwarrior.com

Table of contents

Introduction

We aim to re-evaluate your eating habits, showing you how to fuel your body with the correct nutrition needed to achieve the desired results and also to re-educate you on the fundamentals of weight loss by working on building lean muscle, shifting the focus from calorie counting to achieving long term sustainable results.

Our plan incorporates key micro and macro nutrients essential to your health and well-being, formulated by qualified Personal and Sports Nutritionists.

To make things even simpler, we have put together a comprehensive shopping list, separated into sections you typically find in your favourite grocery store.

Make sure to print this out for your next grocery shopping, and you won't be tempted to give in to endless unhealthy temptations in the store. This list will also give you the added advantage of being able to calculate your weekly food budget, leaving you extra cash left over to splash out on some well deserved TLC.

Disclaimer

We encourage all participants to eat a healthy, well balanced diet to ensure you achieve your desired goal. People with allergies or any food intolerances should endeavour to consult a physician before partaking in this meal plan. We do not make any claims or guarantees about the veracity of the result. Therefore, we do not accept any liabilities therein.

Shopping list

Seasoning
Cracked black peppered
Paprika
Himalayan rock salt
Dried mixed herbs
Cayenne pepper
Cinnamon

Nuts & Seeds
Pumpkin seeds
Almonds
Flaked almonds
Pine nuts
Pistachio nuts

Dairy
Milk
Feta cheese
Low fat soft cheese
Natural/Greek yoghurt 500ml pot x 2
Small block of low fat cheese

Carbohydrates
Wholegrain pasta
Wholegrain rice cakes x 2
Tortilla wraps
Rye bread
White potatoes or baby potatoes
Sweet potato x 5

Shopping list

Fruit & Veg

Bananas x 7
Tomatoes
Mixed salad leaves
Cucumber
Avocado x 3
Aubergine
Courgette x 3
Red onions
Garlic
Chilli
Carrots
Parsnips
Leeks
Celery
Peppers (Red, Yellow & Green) x 5
Mushrooms
Blueberries
Spinach
Spring onions
Grapefruit
Apple x 3
Raspberries
Lemon
Parsley
Cabbage
Broccoli
Frozen peas/vegetables
Lettuce

Shopping list

Tinned Food
Tinned tuna x 2
Tinned Red kidney beans
Tinned chopped tomatoes x 3
Tinned sweetcorn x 1
Tinned chickpeas x 2
Tin of fruit cocktail x 1
Tinned Black eyed beans (if desired)

Protein
Chicken breasts x 6
Whole chicken
Eggs x 7
Lean beef or turkey mince
Smoked salmon
Lean steak
Turkey steaks

Shopping list

Extras
Porridge oats
Honey
Sun dried tomatoes
Olives
Low fat custard x 2 pots
Light mayonnaise
Coconut oil
85% good quality dark chocolate
Vanilla essence
Baking powder
Dried cranberries
Maple syrup (if desired)
Peanut butter
Tomato purée
Reduced salt soy sauce
Hot chocolate
Green Tea
Desiccated coconut
Small pot of sugar free jelly

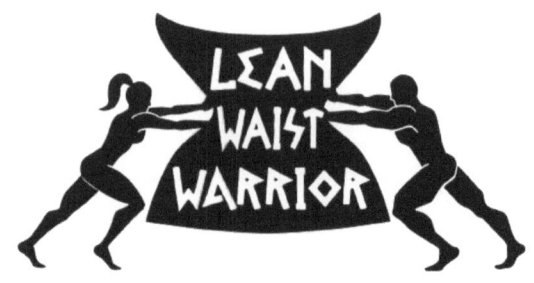

Unleash your inner warrior

Lean Waist Warrior

DAY 1 – Meal Plan

Aim for 2-4L of water daily and replace tea/coffee with Green tea

Day 1

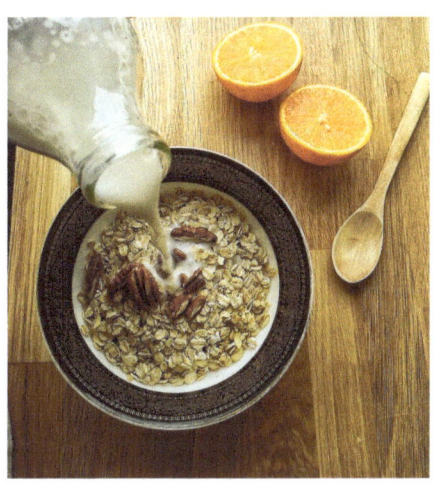

Breakfast

Porridge Oats

*30g of Oats made with water. Sprinkle a handful of pumpkin seeds or almonds, drizzle some honey and finish with a splash of low fat milk.

Day 1

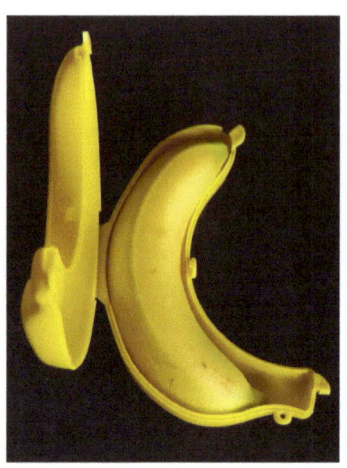

Mid-Morning Snack

One Medium size banana.

Day 1

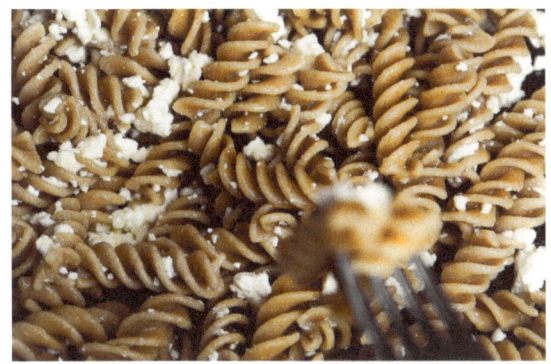

Lunch

Pasta with Greek Salad

*100g of wholegrain Pasta. Slice some fresh tomatoes, lettuce, cucumber, sun dried tomatoes, olives and sprinkle on some crumbled feta cheese.

Day 1

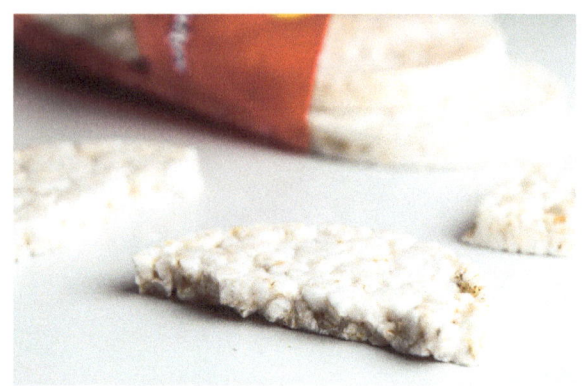

Mid-Afternoon snack

Mix a small tin of tuna, a tablespoon of light mayonnaise, one tablespoon of sweetcorn and season with cracked black pepper. Spread on three wholegrain rice cakes and a few slices of cucumber.

Day 1

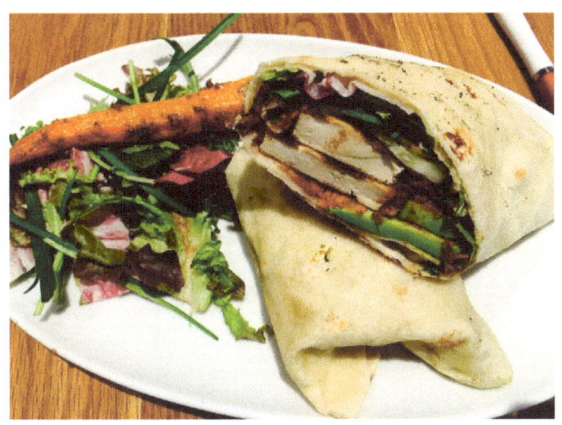

Dinner

Chicken Wraps

*One soft flour tortilla with a tablespoon of low fat soft cheese, 30g skinless chicken breasts, 25g of sweetcorn and a selection of roasted Mediterranean vegetables.

Serve with a mixed side salad. (swap salad dressing for avocado).

Day 1

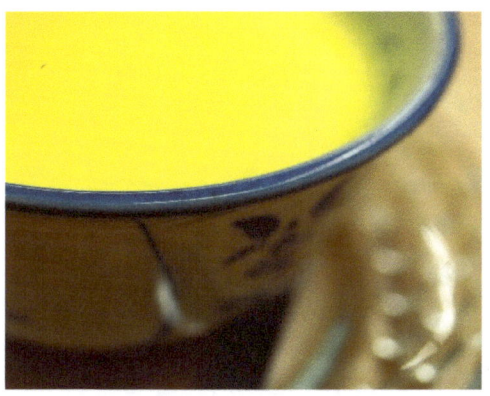

Mid-Evening Snack

One small pot of low fat custard.

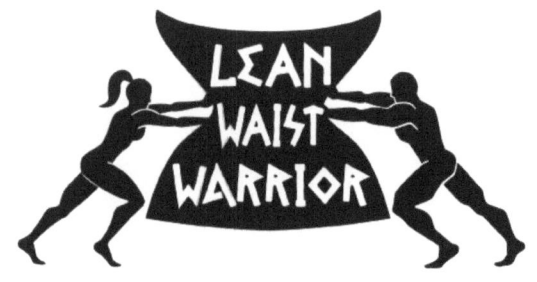

Unleash your inner warrior

Lean Waist Warrior

DAY 2 – Meal Plan

Aim for 2-4L of water daily and replace tea/coffee with Green tea

Day 2

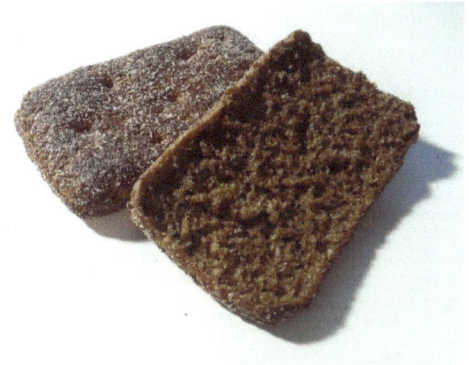

Breakfast

Cheese on toast

*Two slices of rye bread with a tablespoon of low fat soft cheese, half an avocado, sliced tomato and a sliced boiled egg. Season with some paprika and cracked black pepper.

Day 2

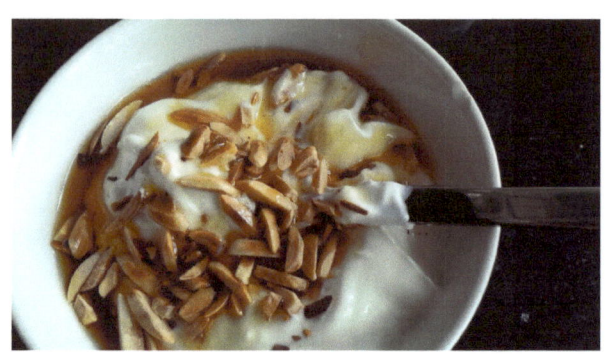

Mid-Morning Snack

125g of natural/Greek yoghurt with honey and flaked almonds.

Day 2

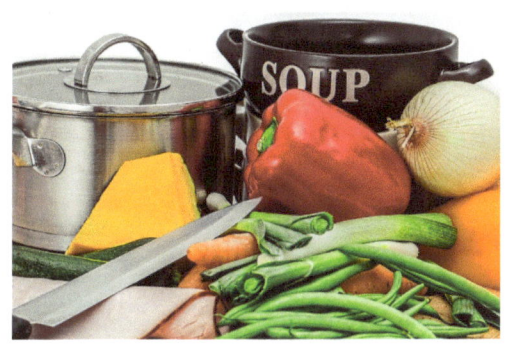

Lunch

Homemade Vegetable Soup

*Chop onions, garlic, chilli & soften in coconut oil.

Add a selection of chopped carrots, parsnips, leeks, celery & 50g of potatoes chopped into chunks.

Add enough water to cover all the contents in the pot. Season with Himalayan rock salt and cracked black pepper as desired.

Day 2

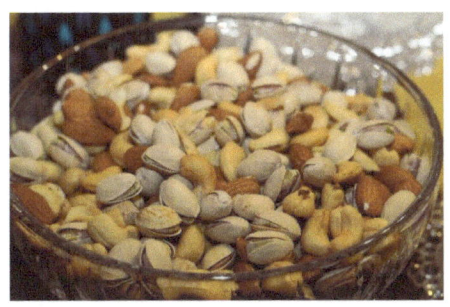

Mid-Afternoon snack

30 pistachio nuts or 15 almonds.

Day 2

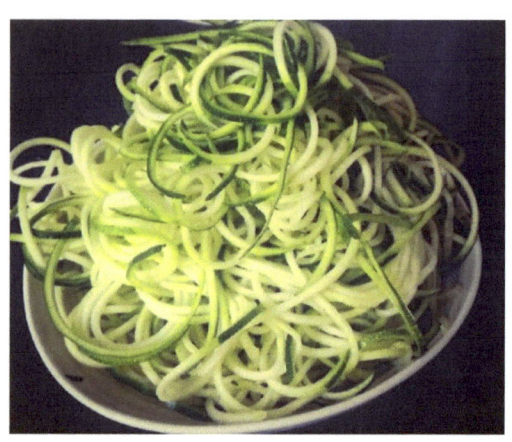

Dinner

Courgetti Bolognese

*Chop onions, garlic, chilli and soften in a tablespoon of coconut oil.

Add 75g of extra lean minced beef/turkey.

Add a tin of chopped tomatoes, half a teaspoon of tomato purée. Add a tin of red kidney beans, chop up a red pepper and mushrooms. Sprinkle with some dried mixed herbs and cracked black pepper. Top with grated low fat cheese.

Replace traditional spaghetti with courgetti (easily done with a potato peeler) and experiment with carrots, courgettes and parsnips.

Day 2

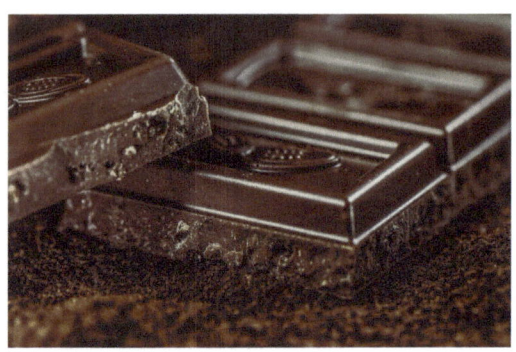

Mid-Evening Snack

2 squares of 85% good quality dark chocolate.

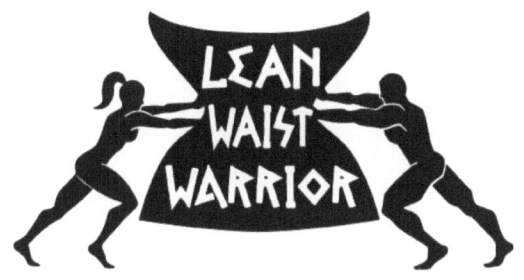

Unleash your inner warrior

Lean Waist Warrior

DAY 3 – Meal Plan

Aim for 2-4L of water daily and replace tea/coffee with Green tea

Day 3

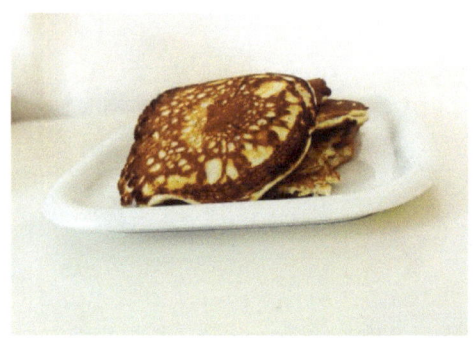

Breakfast

Gluten free pancakes

* Mash 1 medium ripe banana, add two whisked large eggs, a few drops of vanilla essence, half a teaspoon of baking powder, a tablespoon of honey/maple syrup

and some dried cranberries or fresh blueberries.

Cook in coconut oil and serve with some natural/Greek yoghurt and pumpkin seeds as desired.

Day 3

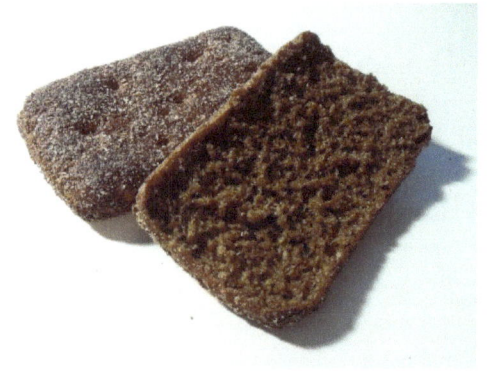

Mid-Morning Snack

One slice of toasted rye bread topped with some smoked salmon, half a mashed avocado and cracked black pepper.

Day 3

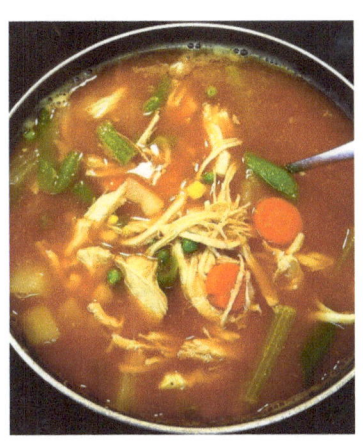

Lunch

Chicken and Vegetable Soup

*Chop onions, garlic, chilli and soften in coconut oil.

Add a selection of chopped carrots, parsnips, leeks, celery, and 50g of potatoes chopped into chunks. Add enough water to cover all the contents in the pot.

Add 25g of cooked chopped chicken. Season with Himalayan rock salt and pepper as desired.

Day 3

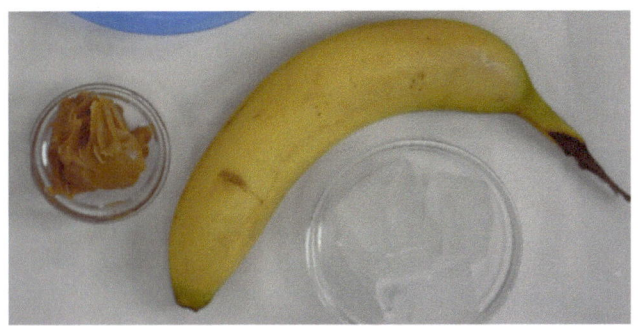

Mid-Afternoon Snack

One medium banana with a teaspoon of peanut butter.

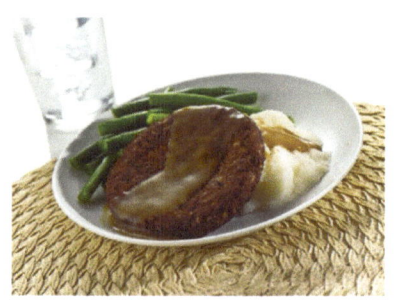

Dinner

Steak and Mashed Potatoes

*4 oz. lean steak, cooked in coconut oil and season with cracked black pepper. Soften a red onion and a handful of spinach in the same pan using the juices of the steak to flavour.

One large sweet potato (baked or mashed), served with black pepper, a crushed garlic clove, and finely chopped spring onions.

Day 3

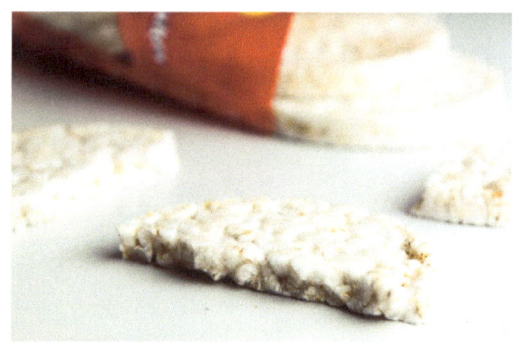

Mid-Evening Snack

Three wholegrain rice cakes with peanut butter and a drizzle of honey.

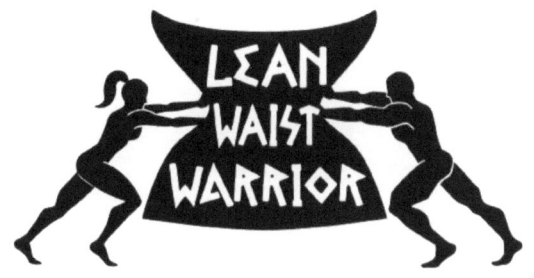

Unleash your inner warrior

Lean Waist Warrior

DAY 4 – Meal Plan

Aim for 2-4L of water daily and replace tea/coffee with Green tea

Day 4

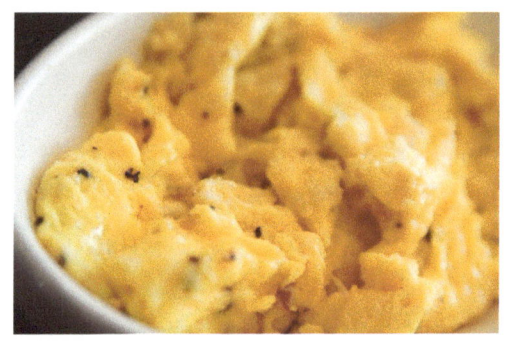

Breakfast

Scrambled Eggs

*Whisk two large eggs and add a splash of milk. Add finely chopped garlic, chilli and half a small onion.

Mix with a few cherry tomatoes cut into quarters, sliced mushrooms, and a few tablespoons of black eye beans/chick peas

Cook in a teaspoon of coconut oil. Season with paprika, Himalayan rock salt and cracked black pepper. Serve with 2 slices of toasted rye bread topped with half a mashed avocado, sprinkled with cayenne pepper.

Day 4

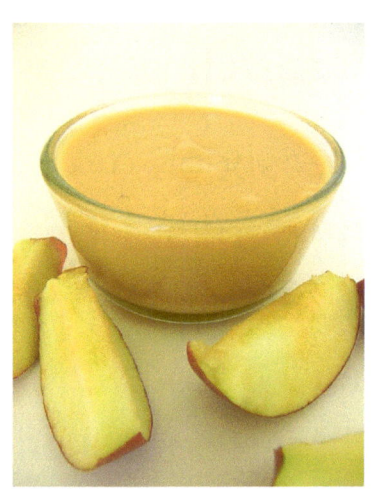

Mid-Morning Snack

One Medium size Apple with two tablespoons of peanut butter.

Day 4

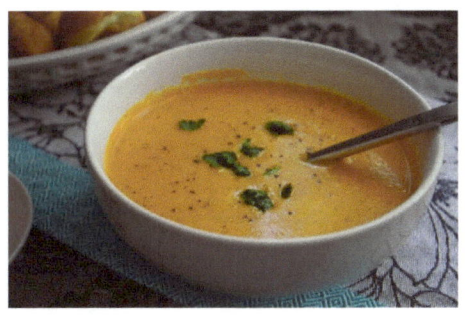

Lunch

Carrot Soup

*Chop onions, garlic, chilli and soften in coconut oil. Add a handful of chopped parsnips, leeks and celery.

Grate 3 or 4 medium carrots and pour in enough water to cover all the contents in the pot. Season with Himalayan rock salt and pepper.

If desired, add to a blender for a smooth finish.

Day 4

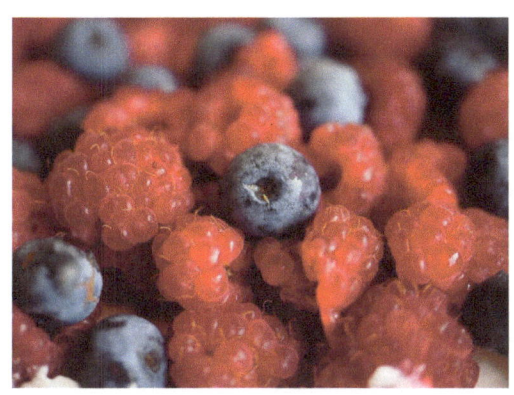

Mid-Afternoon snack

A handful of blueberries and raspberries.

Day 4

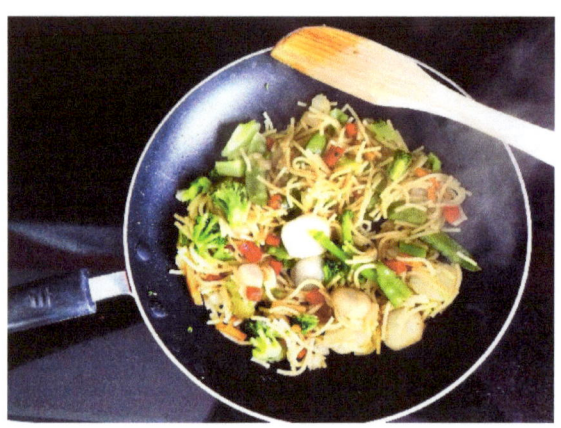

Dinner

Turkey Stir-Fry

*Chop onions, garlic, chilli and soften in coconut oil.

Add a grated carrot, thinly sliced spring onions, peppers, mushrooms.

85g skinless turkey breast strips, a splash of reduced salt soy sauce, and season with a pinch of cracked black pepper. Replace noodles with courgetti (experiment with courgettes, carrots or parsnips).

Day 4

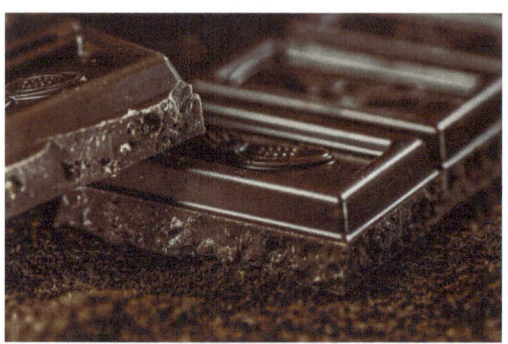

Mid-Evening Snack

1 mug of hot chocolate and 2 squares of 85% good quality dark chocolate.

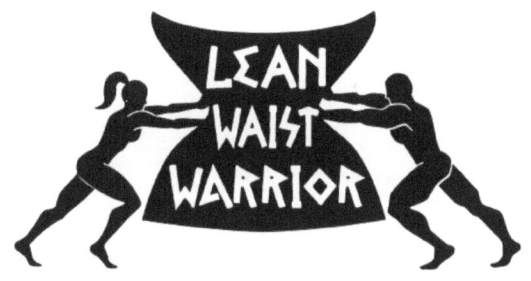

Unleash your inner warrior

Lean Waist Warrior

DAY 5 – Meal Plan

Aim for 2-4L of water daily and replace tea/coffee with Green tea

Day 5

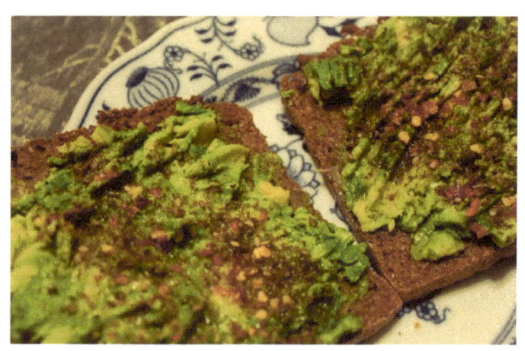

Breakfast

Avocado Toast

*Two slices of toasted rye bread, topped with half a mashed avocado, sliced cherry tomatoes and sprinkle some cayenne pepper and cracked black pepper.

Day 5

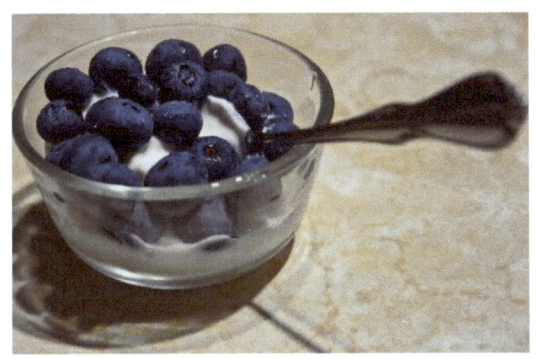

Mid-Morning Snack

100g of natural/Greek yoghurt with a handful of blueberries and a drizzle of honey.

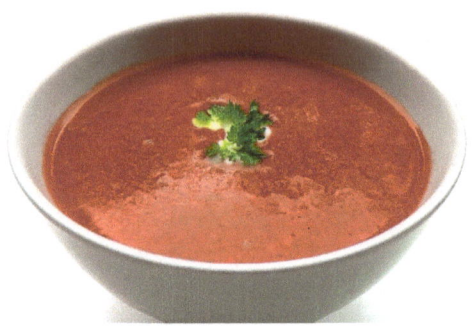

Lunch

Tomato Soup

*Chop onions, garlic, chilli and soften in coconut oil. Add a tin of chopped tomatoes, a handful of chopped fresh cherry tomatoes and a teaspoon of tomato purée.

Stir in some chopped carrots, leeks, and celery. Add enough water to cover all the contents in the pot. Season with Himalayan rock salt and paprika.

For a smooth soup, add the contents to a blender and serve with a spoon of natural/Greek yoghurt and cracked black pepper.

Day 5

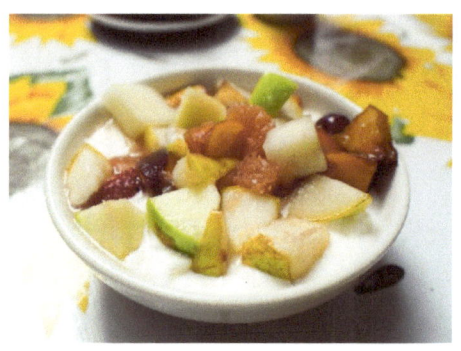

Mid-Afternoon snack

Add a tin of fruit cocktail and fresh grapefruit. Add two tablespoons of natural/Greek yoghurt, drizzle some honey or maple syrup and finish with a sprinkle of cinnamon.

Day 5

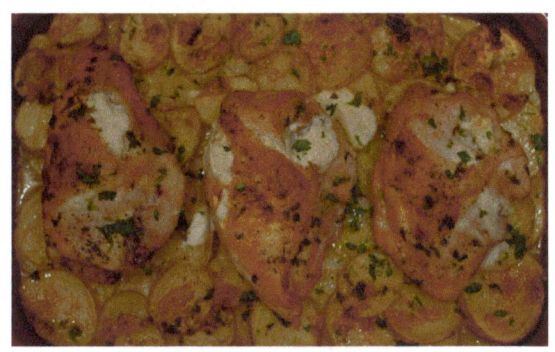

Dinner

Chicken & Potato Bake

*Chop onions, garlic, chilli and soften in coconut oil. Add 50g of chopped chicken breast, a handful of cubed aubergine, courgette, sliced red and yellow pepper.

Season with paprika and cayenne pepper. Toss in a handful of pine nuts and top with two medium sliced sweet potatoes. Finish with a small sprinkle of grated cheese, cracked black pepper and roast in the oven until the sweet potatoes are brown and crispy.

Day 5

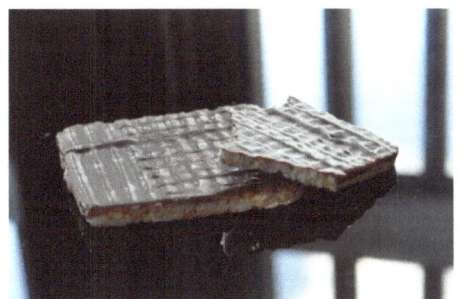

Mid-Evening Snack

Melt 2 squares of 85% dark chocolate and drizzle over three whole grain rice cakes thinly spread with peanut butter.

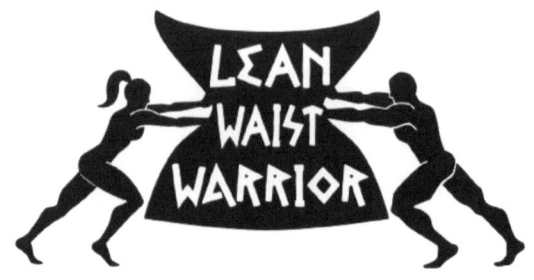

Unleash your inner warrior

Lean Waist Warrior

DAY 6 – Meal Plan

Aim for 2-4L of water daily and replace tea/coffee with Green tea

Day 6

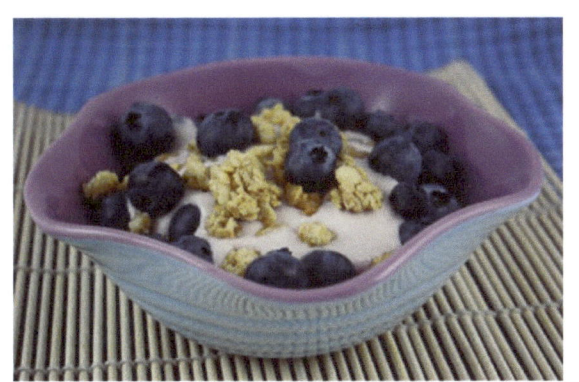

Breakfast

Granola yoghurt

*Add a large handful of oats and two tablespoons of desiccated coconut to a hot pan, with coconut oil until lightly golden.

Mix with 150g of natural/Greek yoghurt, a handful of blueberries and pumpkin seeds. Sprinkle with cinnamon and drizzle some maple syrup.

Day 6

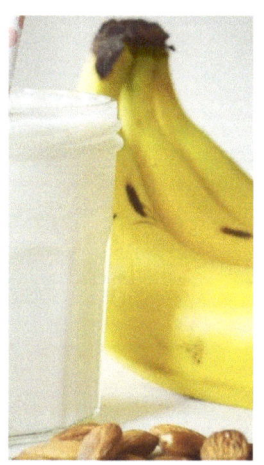

Mid-Morning Snack

A medium banana with a handful of almonds.

Day 6

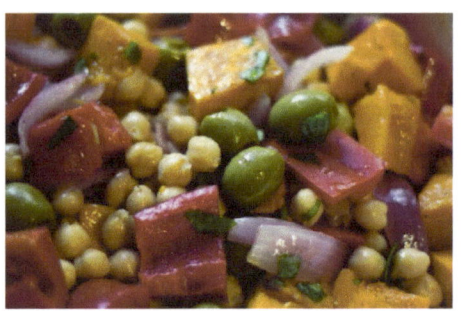

Lunch

Chickpea & Roasted Pepper Salad

*Add mixed salad leaves, sliced cucumber, cherry tomato halves, grated carrot, finely chopped red onion, spring onions, half an avocado, a tin of chickpeas, 50g of crumbled feta cheese and two tablespoons of sweetcorn.

Roast 2 medium red peppers in the oven until they have softened. Once cooled, chop the peppers and add to the salad. Season with some freshly squeezed lemon, chopped parsley and cracked black pepper.

Day 6

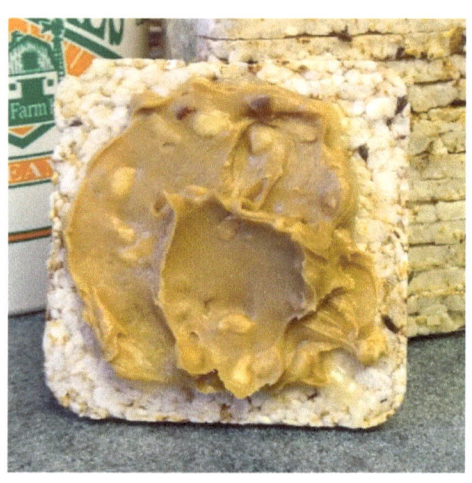

Mid-Afternoon snack

Three wholegrain rice cakes with peanut butter.

Day 6

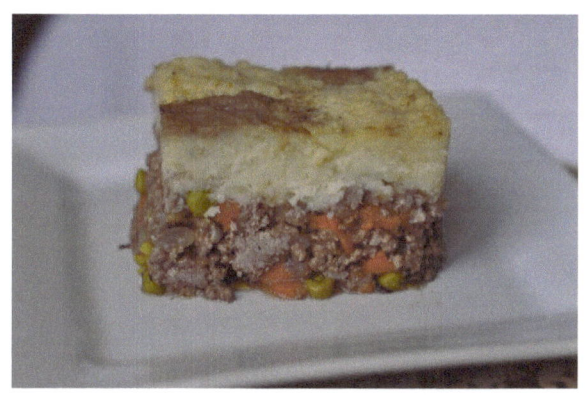

Dinner

Shepherds Pie

*Chop onions, garlic, chilli and soften in a tablespoon of coconut oil. Add 75g of extra lean minced beef/turkey.

Add a tin of chopped tomatoes, half a teaspoon of tomato purée.

Chop two carrots, a red pepper and mushrooms and add to the sauce. Sprinkle with some dried mixed herbs and cracked black pepper. Top with two mashed sweet potatoes and roast in the oven until crispy.

Day 6

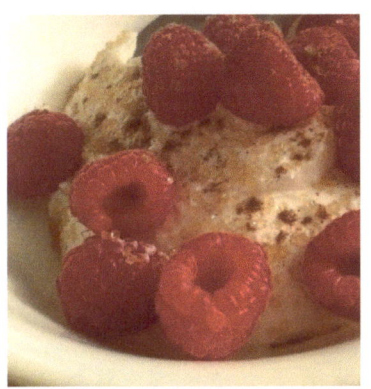

Mid-Evening Snack

100g of natural/Greek yoghurt with raspberries and a square of 85% good quality dark chocolate grated on top.

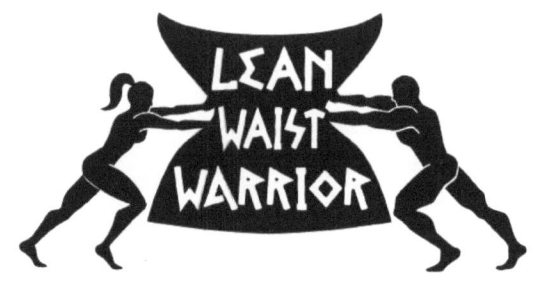

Unleash your inner warrior

Lean Waist Warrior

DAY 7 – Meal Plan

Aim for 2-4L of water daily and replace tea/coffee with Green tea

Day 7

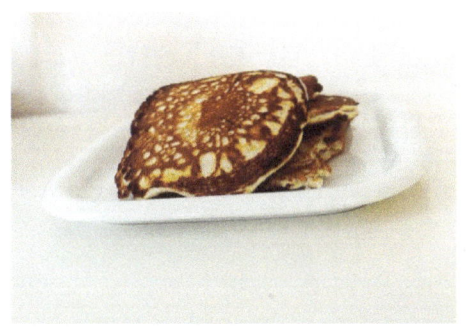

Breakfast

Gluten free pancakes

*Mash one medium ripe banana, add two whisked large eggs, a few drops of vanilla essence, half a teaspoon of baking powder.

One tablespoon of honey/maple syrup and some dried cranberries or fresh blueberries.

Cook in coconut oil and serve with some natural/Greek yoghurt and seeds as desired.

Day 7

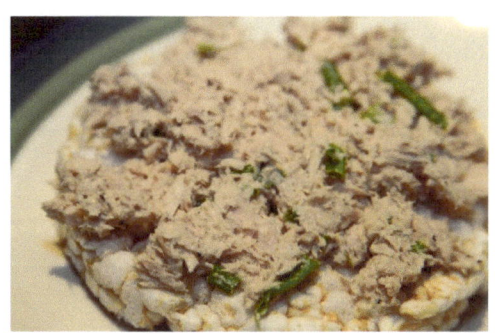

Mid-Morning Snack

Mix a small tin of tuna, a tablespoon of light mayo, one tablespoon of sweetcorn and season with cracked black pepper. Spread on three wholegrain rice cakes and a few slices of cucumber.

Day 7

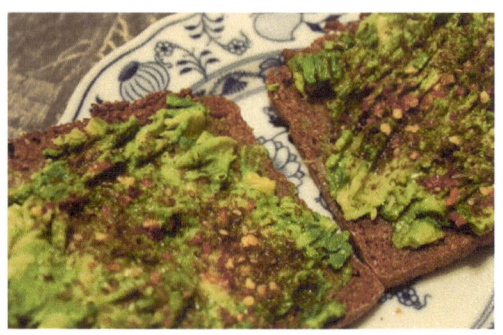

Lunch

Avocado Toast

*Two slices of toasted rye bread, topped with half a mashed avocado, sliced cherry tomatoes and sprinkle some cayenne pepper and cracked black pepper.

Day 7

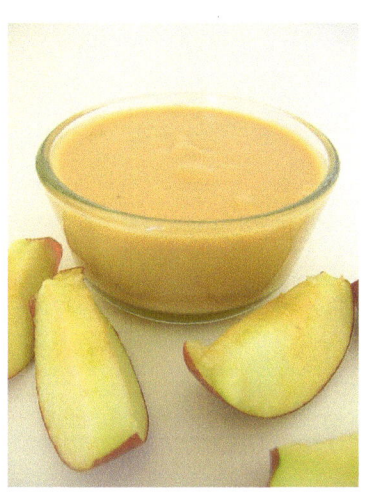

Mid-Afternoon snack

An apple with peanut butter.

Day 7

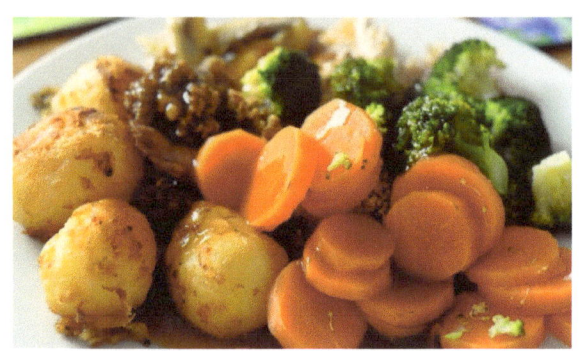

Dinner

Sunday Roast – Enjoy!

*Roast chicken, served with two large boiled potatoes or home made roast potatoes or baby potatoes with the skins on.

Boil two carrots, a handful of cabbage, broccoli and frozen peas. Serve with some reduced salt gravy granules.

Day 7

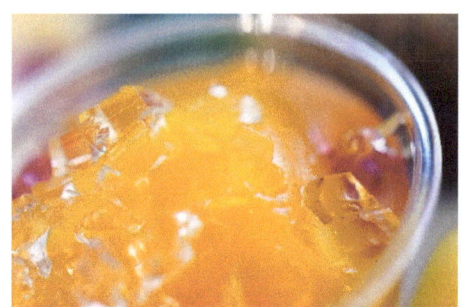

Mid-Evening Snack

A small pot of sugar free jelly with small pot of low fat custard.

STAY STRONG, WARRIOR!

Other Books From Author

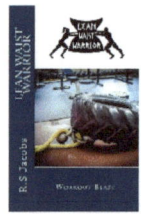

Lean Waist Warrior

Workout Blast

Available on Amazon

www.ingramcontent.com/pod-product-compliance
Lightning Source LLC
Chambersburg PA
CBHW040321010626
45792CB00024B/2081